PALEO 30 DAY CHALLENGE

A Beginner's Guide To Diet, Rapid Weight Loss & Natural Living.

Habits, Tips & Paleo Recipes For Success

CASEY CROFT

ISBN-13: 9781521198803

DISCLAIMER

This book is not intended as a substitute for the medical advice of physicians. You should consult a physician before embarking on any kind of diet or exercise program, especially if you have any known pre-existing medical conditions.

This book is agnostic to food allergies or intolerances and is written with the assumption that the reader does not suffer from these conditions. If you do have food allergies, please do not deviate from any traditional approaches you current follow for those mentioned within this book without consulting your medical professional.

No liability is accepted for any illness or injury that results from following the strategies or recipes in this book.

CONTENTS

PART ONE: 30 DAY PALEO INTRODUCTION

Many books are available that aim to help you adopt a Paleo lifestyle. However, there is more to this than simply a diet. It is not enough to know the allowed and banned foods. For many people, a highly processed Western diet (sometimes referred to as the Standard American Diet, or SAD) is the only thing they've ever known. Coupled with a sedentary, office-based lifestyle, adopting the Paleo method is a challenge for most people.

This book is designed to do more than tell you what to eat. It is designed to give you the information you need to not only complete the 30 day challenge but also continue with it well beyond that first month. It contains proven strategies to help you make a change that is more to do with lifestyle than a quick win, temporary diet. It requires a radical shift in thinking to move towards a healthier lifestyle that has countless nutritional benefits over one that revolves around sugary, refined carbohydrates as well as other processed foods. In fact, understanding why to go Paleo and the difficulties you may experience is so important that the information on what you can eat doesn't appear until chapter five. There are fundamental lessons that must be understood first.

For many people, the cost of healthcare is untenable. An undisputed fact is that putting excessive quantities of toxins into our bodies leads to a whole range of medical conditions. The spectrum ranges from mild intolerances to catastrophic, even fatal, organ failure. The best way to reduce the risks associated with the modern lifestyle is to return to the way of living that sustained the human race from its infancy. A diet that is more about gaining nutrition than making profits for large companies churning food from factories to plate.

This book will also address that many of the additives these companies put in foods are designed to be highly addictive. Sugar, modified fats, salt and genetically modified material create cravings for more of the food we should avoid. To pretend you will not feel cravings and withdrawal from these items means you are likely to fail if you think that switching takeout for home cooked meat and vegetables is purely a change in cooking choices.

Because of this, throughout the book you will find modified Paleo alternatives. Whilst this deviates from the challenge in the strictest sense, it has two positive effects. The first is that it allows for people with certain dietary requirements to make smarter choices without knowingly causing possible health implications. Secondly, for those people who have consumed nothing but pre-packaged, heavily modified foods for a prolonged period to wean themselves off this food without too many side effects. After thirty days of success on the modified diet, it will then be possible to repeat the process with a full implementation of the Paleo way of life.

Similarly, it means knowing the right questions to ask when dining out at restaurants, or participating in other social occasions. It can be done effectively and most establishments are more than happy to meet any dietary requirements. Understanding the dos and don'ts of Paleo food will help you articulate these requirements more clearly to ensure you get only wholesome, clean food on your plate, rather than any nasty surprises.

You'll also notice that the majority of recipes in this

book do not contain any portion sizes or weights. This is because the Paleo diet is not a calorie-controlled diet of the kind that has been popular over the past fifty years. Instead, it is about eating for your bodies needs and learning to recognize its own internal control systems again. Without modified and addictive substances creating harmful feedback loops in your biochemistry, you will earn to consume the amount of food that is right for *you*, not a pre-ordained calorie restricted choice that meets someone else's needs.

CHAPTER ONE: WHY PALEO?

This book has not been written from the perspective of a doctor, nutritionist or biochemist. It is not a science book that will explain the fundamentals of how the body processes food. However, it will give you enough information to understand why a Paleo diet could work for you and what you need to do implement it. If you are curious to find out more, especially at a deeper biochemical level, there are many great resources out there to help you do that. Most people, however, simply need to know the basics- enough information to get them started.

So what do people mean when they talk about a Paleo diet? It refers to the diet consumed by our biological ancestors back in the Paleolithic era. This can be defined as 50,000 to 10,000 years ago, although the Paleolithic era began much earlier than that. What is key about this time period for our purposes is that humans were closely evolved to the level of our current species and had started to use basic tools. This led to a rudimentary level of food preparation that we can mimic today, but was not advanced enough to include those items that are classified as processed. If it was available and you could pick it, kill it, cook it or make it, then it is available for your consumption on the Paleo diet.

There are several versions of the Paleolithic Diet available, requiring different levels of dedication and intensity. The basic principle is simple: would I have eaten this in my cave 50,000 years ago? There is an emphasis on meat, vegetables, fruits, nuts and seeds to make up the energy and nutrient requirements for the human body. Any food groups commonly included in the modern Western diet were only introduced by farming (from approximately 15,000-10,000 BC onwards) are excluded.

The exact details of these foods will be covered later. First, we need to explain the benefits of them and, more importantly, the dangers of the alternatives.

So what are the advantages of doing this? Perhaps it is more useful for people to see the disadvantages of the alternative. The Paleo diet, although providing you with ambulant amounts of food, will nevertheless feel restrictive to many people who are not used to controlling what they eat this way. At best, they may have attempted calorie restriction as a weight loss method. This is not the same as a Paleo diet as it does not, by default, eliminate the harmful chemicals being added to the body by processed foods.

Processed foods come heavily laden with two ingredients that are toxic to our body in large quantities. These are sugars and certain fats. For many years, fat was made the enemy and with it the low fat revolution took place. Stores were filled with convenient, low fat alternatives to everything. However, with the natural fat taken out, it was replaced with either man-made fats or added sugar. Often, it contained both.

The increase in obesity rates of people consuming these low fat foods, especially as part of a calorie-controlled lifestyle is the first warning that a deviation away from the Paleo diet and into a modern Western lifestyle is harmful to the body. Although we have also become more sedentary, it is unlikely that lack of exercise alone can account for the statistical shift towards obesity and poor health. Therefore, we must understand what is contained in these processed foods and, as a result, how they are destroying our bodies from the inside.

Let's take a look first at man-made fats. The most obvious example are trans fats, introduced originally as a healthy alternative to saturated fats, which occur naturally in many Paleo foods, such as meat. Given the link between excess saturated fat and high cholesterol, trans fats were devised as a replacement that could be added to products such as margarine and cooking oils.

Like many man-made ingredients that are added to processed foods, only rudimentary checks are ever performed before they are authorized for human consumption. In this particular scenario, it has since been discovered, years after it was introduced, to not only increase the dangerous types of cholesterol (known as 'bad' cholesterol) but also *decreased* the 'good' cholesterol. There is a common misconception that all cholesterol is bad. However, good cholesterol plays an important role in removing the bad cholesterol from your system, taking it back to the liver so it can be removed from the body rather than deposited elsewhere. As a result, 'good' cholesterol is essential in reducing your risk of heart attack or stroke.

You *can* consume too much saturated fat, especially

in a world where meats are readily available. However, instead of advising the reduction in high-saturated foods, in seeking an alternative to a way of living that had allowed man to evolve successfully over many thousands of years, the chemical, lab created alternatives exacerbated the problem. Natural fats should be, and always were until the last century, a significant part of our diet. Other carnivorous and omnivorous mammals do not avoid fat and neither should we. Seeking unnatural fats is not the alternative.

The second reason to avoid processed food and adopt a Paleo lifestyle is added sugars. Like saturated fats, sugars occur naturally in food and are an essential part of the human diet. However, when consumed in excess, they can become deadly. This is a fact that is only recently being acknowledged by the medical establishment. After years of creating low fat food laden with a sugar alternative, nearly all food companies are also resistant to revealing how dangerous this is.

Like trans fats, the chemistry and its consequences are often hidden from consumer view. This is deliberate. It allows the promotion of so-called 'natural sugars' as healthy. However, this is not the case. For our ancestors, fruit did not occur in abundance. Commercial orchards create the impression of such, but fruit trees were widely interspersed. They needed to be, as they had to compete for naturally occurring soil nutrients. Today, intensive farming means these nutrients are artificially added to the soil, allowing mass crops production.

But this is not what our metabolic system developed for.

When talking about sugar, most people think of it in two ways. Either as a single entity (for example, the white granular sugar) or, if they know some limited chemistry, as 'glucose'. On nutrition composition labels, you will only ever see - and even then not always - sugar given as a subset of carbohydrate. In fact, these simplistic terms aren't helpful and mask the real danger of eating a Western processed diet rather than Paleo.

Processed sugar, the white stuff as we know it, is actually made of two molecules: glucose and fructose. I won't get too technical here, but fructose as an energy source is used differently to all other carbohydrate. It is this biochemical limitation that makes it dangerous in large quantities.

Sugar is a great energy source. It, along with protein and natural fats, form the backbone of the energy supply we as humans use to stay alive. Glucose is our primary energy source for a good reason. Our bodies have developed to use it efficiently. Our brains require it to think and grow. Our body can also store it as energy, a requirement from Paleolithic times when meals did not occur with predictable regularity three times a day. Those stores allowed us to burn energy long after our last meal until we could find the next one. Our metabolic system carefully monitors glucose levels and shifts our biochemistry in response. It does the complex chemical calculations deep within the primitive part of our brain and works out how much we consumed, how much we have left and therefore whether or not we feel hungry.

Fructose, as a molecule, bypasses this clever system. It does so for a very good reason, one that is deeply rooted in the Paleo diet. As stated earlier, commercial farming gives the impression that fruit was a readily available food source when in reality it was scarce. Nevertheless, it was still a fantastic food source, laden with easy energy in the form of fructose and macro- and micronutrients that allow for optimum running of the machine known as the human body. Back then, it was more concerned with survival.

By removing fructose from the metabolic feedback loop, early humans could literally gorge themselves when they came across a fruit tree. Nomadic by nature, the combination of finding a tree and it being in perfect season was the Paleo equivalent of hitting a gold mine.

The body metabolized the other ingredients, but fructose is only metabolized by the liver. Any fructose, whether from eating an apple or from an entire box of cookies, can only go to the liver. The liver takes what it needs to survive and then converts the remainder to fatty acids for storage.

That's right. If you can't use the energy you consume as fructose then it turns to fat. If you can't use that within a few days, it continues to circulate the blood stream, being deposited in arteries, liver or stored for long-term use. Not a problem for our ancestors, but with a constant supply of sugar added to our modern processed food, the majority of people are guaranteed to consume more than they can burn.

The second danger too is that because it bypasses the metabolic system used by all other food groups, the brain is unaware of it. This means it is unable to include it in the calculations is makes to determine if we are hungry or full.

Perfect for our food deprived ancestors. A recipe for disaster for us.

This is why calorie controlled diets that allow processed foods often fail. Fat is stripped, sugar is added and because your body is blissfully unaware of half of that sugar, people feel hungry. In the past two hundred years, the average American yearly sugar consumption increased from approximately 6lbs to a peak of over 105lbs per year in 1999. It has reduced slightly since then, but still hovers around 100lbs. That is a significant dietary change in a supposedly more health conscious and aware time.

With new research becoming available each day about the impacts of highly processed food on overall health, the food and exercise combination of the Paleo movement gains increasing relevance and value. Years of modified fat, high sugar, packaged food combined with reduced exercise levels are now being linked to the following conditions:

- Heart diseases
- Fatty liver disease
- Metabolic syndrome
- Pancreatic diseases

- Type II diabetes
- Several types of cancer
- Female fertility problems
- Autism
- Alzheimer's disease

These are all chronic conditions that have risen dramatically since the Western diet has moved from fresh to packaged convenience foods. The Paleo diet could reduce the risk or completely prevent these health issues. For those already dealing with the onset of these terrible illnesses, making the change to a way of life back to what nature intended could help lessen the symptoms and, in some cases, even reverse the damage done.

CHAPTER TWO: ADVANTAGES OF PALEO OVER OTHER DIETS

With so many alternatives, why choose Paleo over other diets?

The first thing to note is that Paleo is more than a 'diet'. Although it involves making a conscious effort regarding food choice, it is not about restricting the amount you can eat. It is not about swapping tasty food and happiness in exchange for being thin, which is what most people associate with the dieting concept.

Instead, changing the thought process around Paleo from 'diet' to 'positive lifestyle change' prevents these negative connotations underpinning your motivations and rooting the diet in failure. Along with our metabolism, one of the things that developed during the Paleo years was the awareness that we need to protect ourselves from pain and unhappiness. Therefore, if we think that our food choices will make us hungry and miserable then once the initial burst of motivation wears off then a relapse towards packaged foods will happen very quickly.

Paleo is not a diet. It is a new habit to build a stronger, healthier you.

There are many positives about eating only Paleo food, rather than convenience foods filled with chemical additives and enhancers, but the underlying foundation is that your metabolic system will return to normal. That means that the hormones that let you know if you are hungry or sated will begin to tell the truth. Eating food based on genuine hunger means that you do not have to worry about calorie counting or portion control once you have completed the 30 day challenge on this diet. You consume the energy and nutrients your body needs and it tells you to stop eating. You eat when you become hungry again. It is beautiful in its simplicity.

Still tempted by other options? Here's how they stack up.

Paleo or calorie control (this includes so-called 'points' systems)?

For the past fifty years, diets have been developed around nothing more than controlling your calorie intake. These have been promoted by celebrities to sell the idea that a multinational corporation can make you thin if you buy their products and pay to attend their weekly sessions and classes.

In recent years, this extreme restriction and control has been made more appealing to those who have already tried (and failed) the approach by building in cheat days and artificially sweetened products but it does not change the long term success ratios. It can include restricting your food to a very narrow group that contains multiple artificial chemicals anyway.

People lose weight on these diets, especially in the beginning. A calorie deficit will always lead to weight loss. People give up the diet when they reach an inevitable and demoralizing plateau. From our Paleo standpoint, this is basic and obvious evolution. When food was scarce, the human metabolic system slowed down to conserve energy and run more efficiently. It stores each energy unit it can to prolong the chances of survival until the next food source appears.

Following the Paleo approach uses this knowledge to much better purpose than simply eating small amounts of food and starving yourself thin.

From a health perspective, skinny due to calorie

deficiency doesn't automatically equate to healthy. Men in particular may lose weight but struggle to maintain muscle mass and tone. The low-calorie branded products contain significant amounts of chemical preservatives and added sugars that do long term damage to organs that you can't see. It is far better to eat Paleo and know you are building a strong, healthy body.

Paleo or low carb?

A common alternative to Paleo is ultra low carbohydrate. Made popular by the Atkins Diet, it eliminates all carbohydrates in favor of protein and fat. It produces very fast weight loss and muscle gain definitely, especially when combined with intense training. Because of this, the low carb diet has long been the choice of the ultra-healthy and those into serious fitness. It is very effective.

However, the body was designed to work at its most efficient by utilizing glucose. Our primary food sources contain complex carbohydrates, making the diet hard to maintain in the long term. A simple, high carbohydrate meal by mistake can lead to dramatic bloating and water retention.

Ultra low carb makes the body work defensively, in a similar way to starvation. Without available glucose from food, the body will first use its most readily available internal energy in the form of glycogen. This is another precaution that dates back from the Paleo lifestyle. This easy energy exists to sustain us through times when food is scarce. Low carb manipulates the body from its original purpose. This is the opposite of what Paleo is trying to do.

It creates a false sense of weight loss. Glycogen is stored by binding it to water. When a sudden restriction in carbohydrate occurs, much of the sudden weight loss is nothing more than the shedding of water to release this glycogen for use. It is the body's natural function to attempt to store it. So the slightest deviation from the low carb diet will cause those carbohydrates to be instantly put back into muscle storage, along with the water retention required to do so. People who sustain the low carb diet at this level can see a weight increase of up to 5lbs on the scale after a single day including carbohydrates.

It is, of course, at this point where many people become depressed and confused by the sudden change and a pattern of old habits and unhealthy eating returns as the body again craves the food it is missing.

Longer term, when completely deprived of carbohydrates, the body goes into a state known as ketosis. This is a simple, short-term Paleolithic survival method. Longer term, it has been known to have implications of its own, such as sustained damage to vital organs including the liver and kidneys.

Paleo does not eliminate carbohydrates and therefore avoids these dramatic swings in weight or long term health complications.

Paleo or the 'Whole Food' diet

There is often a lot of confusion around the differences between Paleo diets and a 'whole food' approach. This is understandable, as they both emphasize a way of eating that is vastly different from the convenience food, anything goes approach of the modern Western lifestyle.

With an increase in popularity and therefore an abundance of information, it is clear that there are multiple variations of both approaches, which adds an additional layer of confusion.

The whole foods diet is, however, generally

considered to be more restrictive than Paleo. If you wanted to create 'cheat versions' of modern food using only allowed, unprocessed foods, then Paleo does not discourage you from doing so. In comparison, the whole foods approach has a stronger focus on distancing yourself from those modern foods altogether. It is more of a back to basics approach, not just in terms of food choices, but also in food thinking.

Whereas Paleo eliminates by food group, whole food diets frequently exclude partial groups. For example, dairy isn't allowed, but clarified butter is. This is not arbitrary, but can still be confusing and limiting for some people.

So a strict, whole food diet and accompanying mindset shift can be considered as the next extreme from Paleo. For someone beginning their journey to a better, healthier way of living, you will probably find Paleo enough of a challenge during these first thirty days. Consider whole foods at some point in the future, when your current bad food habits and desires have become a thing of the past.

Hopefully that has provided some insight into how Paleo is often the better alternative to other diets out there. As well as issues of long-term sustainability, the benefits of excluding artificial ingredients and focusing on natural ones are clear.

CHAPTER THREE: ADDITIVES AND ADDICTIONS

The biggest difficulty you will encounter when attempting a 30 day Paleo diet challenge is not knowing which foods to eat and how to cook them. That is a common misconception that people make about the difficulties in switching to a Paleo lifestyle.

In fact, the real difficulty comes from your body's response to the removal of artificial additives and chemicals that you have been putting into your body up until that point. Modern food feels like an addiction to many people. But it hasn't always been that way. In fact, food addiction is a relatively new concept and only began to appear shortly after the move away from home cooked, natural meals towards pre-packaged convenience foods.

Recent studies have discovered that one of the main added ingredients to convenience foods, sugar, is as addictive as crack cocaine. Because it is an essential nutrient, salt works in the same way. Given that back in Paleo times, salt was hard to find in the same way as sugar. As a result, our bodies became hardwired to enjoy it to make sure we ate it when we found it.

Unlike recreational drugs, both legal and illegal, salt and sugar are not a conscious choice to make if eating modern processed food. Both have a high probability of being added to anything pre-packaged, even if it is a food you don't associate with being particularly sweet or salty.

Instead, we blindly feed the addiction that has been hardwired for survival. Except now that both of these things are cheap and easily available, the balance has tipped too far the other way. It becomes an unhealthy dependency and one which makes us drawn to the food that gives us the biggest hits. When you choose to go Paleo, you are also making the decision to break an addiction.

Chances are, you won't realize how strong that addiction is until you test it. The problem won't be with the food you can eat, but a psychological and physiological craving for the food you can't.

Mapping the brain shows that when we consume salt, sugar and some fats, pleasure centers light up in response. Over time and repeated activity, these pleasure centers demand the salt and sugar. When you hardwire this natural high and combine it with the chemical disruption of your metabolism, the impact is intense and profound. It also explains why the modern Western diet encourages over-consumption, even though we know on an intellectual level that we are not in a food shortage. Our intellectual brain comes second to the strength of our Paleo brain.

Weight loss is a key goal for many people who embark on the Paleo diet. It is precisely because of these addictive additives that they need to. We can all recognize the foods that are heavily laden with artificial sugars, salts and preservatives. They are the foods that we continue to eat, even as our stomachs begin to bloat with food. They create that craving, 'still hungry' feeling, even though your tightening clothes let you know you've already had enough.

With this intensity of addiction, it is vital to have a strategy in place to help you through this. In the same way that Alcoholics Anonymous provides a support framework of tools and people to help with the worst of the cravings, you can prepare yourself for the short-term pain of withdrawal. The long-term benefits are certainly worth it.

Do you really want to go Paleo?

Now you know that you're addicted to modern food, do you really want to go Paleo? Ask yourself if you are prepared to make more than a dietary change. Your willpower will be tested when craving for processed food begins. Like any other addiction, it will not go away without a fight. So to prepare yourself for the physical responses of withdrawal, you will need to have a good reason to keep going. Knowing this before you start statistically gives you a greater chance of completing 30 days of the Paleo lifestyle. More importantly, it will keep you going long after that first month has finished.

Weight loss itself may not be enough. It is the most common factor that causes people to seek out a new diet. The Paleo approach, if you stick to it for 30 days, will almost guarantee weight loss success.

But what happens after 60 days? Or 90 days? Or however long it takes until you become happy with your new weight? Surrounded by food temptation everywhere, if weight loss alone is your goal, then it will be easy to retreat back to processed foods. Small quantities at first, without any noticeable weight gain or side effects. But as the addiction takes hold again behind the scenes, it won't take long before all good intentions are gone and your Paleo lifestyle is over. Weight gain and the associated health risks return as a result.

Symptoms of addiction and the effects of withdrawal

Cravings for off limit foods will be the most obvious symptom of addiction. The breakfast pastry. The soda with lunch. Take out after a long day at the office. The convenience of grabbing these foods will pair up with a strong desire for them.

The level of cravings varies for everyone. It is not merely a sign of your willpower or commitment. It can be based on your gender, genetic predisposition, racial origins and the quantities of process foods you have consumed. It will vary dependent on whether the change to a Western modern diet occurred only in adulthood or whether it is the diet you have followed since birth.

These symptoms are similar to the so-called 'low carb flu' experienced by athletes and body builders switching from carbohydrates to protein as their primary fuel. This is because some of the root causes are the same. The removal of carbohydrates includes many that have been heavily processed and modified.

Common side effects you may experience during the first ten days of Paleo:

- Headache
- Loss of concentration
- Flu-like symptoms
- Trembling
- Insomnia
- Mood swings
- Exhaustion
- Low grade anxiety

When you look at the list, you will see these side effects are common to any withdrawal process. It is the body's way of coercing you back towards addiction, by making the alternatives painful. Most 30 day challenge and diet books will not warn you of this. That is why so many people fail in the early days of switching to Paleo. They claim that it doesn't work. Or that it is too complicated to follow. But armed with this knowledge, it is possible to meet these challenges head on when they appear. This will increase your odds of success by a significant amount.

Breaking addiction - beyond willpower

Understanding that this is more than eating food but actually changing your body's relationship with it on an emotional and physiological level is a greater way to avoid failure. There are a few key, proactive steps you can take that will mean that once you begin the 30 day challenge, you will not be relying on willpower to keep going.

First, ask yourself this simple question: have I successfully quit any other addiction before? It doesn't matter how mild or serious. It could be caffeine, smoking, alcohol or candy. If you've had any degree of success, then think back to how you did it.

Some people have the greatest success when they remove something from their life completely. There are no cheat days, no excuses. All temptation is removed and the process begins cold turkey. This is a from day one lifestyle change. This is the method often used by alcoholics attending a program. The number of successive days entirely sober is a key monitoring tool.

Others have more success by using the reduction

method. This is the method very often used when someone is deciding to quit smoking. From a pack a day to half a pack, then down to five, then the one after dinner only, then patches to beat the craving. It can feel like a longer process, but it works for many people. Long-term success, as with anything, is more important that 30 days followed by a relapse.

Take the time to think about this, because it really is a personal choice. The more you can adjust the process to work for you, the more benefit you will see. It will also make it feel like more of a conscious choice. More than willpower, free will is an enabling emotion that will allow you to approach the 30 day challenge feeling in control from the start.

The start date is important. If you're about to embark on a week of travel, then do not attempt to start the 30 day challenge. Until you are confident in your own behaviors and the correct foods to ask for, you will not be able to order correctly and will therefore fail straight away. It is important for your body and for your psychology to get the first few days working well. Success spurs more success.

Similarly, try to pick a week clear of social events. Although this isn't always possible with the modern busy lifestyle, it is still important to try. Again, it is about avoiding temptation. It is also about avoiding peer pressure. Even the closest of friends will attempt subtle sabotage if you are making a positive life change and they are not. If all your friends happen to be following the Paleo lifestyle, then go for it. That changes it from a social occasion to a support network and that is entirely different

Once you've taken the time to review, then choose a day and stick to it. Monday is the obvious choice, but it doesn't have to be. The key is to make a decision and commit. Once it is locked in, then you know it will be time to begin your new and healthier way of living.

Final warning - you don't actually live in a cave

This book is designed to help you through the 30 day Paleo challenge. However, this kind of lifestyle change extends for most people into a different way of living. Although it is a conscious decision to change the way you eat, you cannot change the rest of the world around you.

If the 30 day challenge is a resounding success, then that doesn't mean you will never eat in a non-Paleo way again. There are many hardcore Paleo followers out there who have been following the diet for years, if not decades. The majority of them build in 'cheat' days. This is to allow for the times when external circumstances mean eat Western or eat nothing.

I mention this not to encourage you to do so. I am merely highlighting that it happens so that anyone entirely new to the diet doesn't assume that a single instance of failure spells the end of your Paleo change. Of course it doesn't. The modern western diet has flourished because it works so well alongside the current world we live in. Its convenience will always be a temptation when you are tired or had a bad day.

The key to implementing Paleo over the longer term is not to make sure you never fall. It is to make sure you don't stay down when you do.

The highly addictive quality of the additives in mass produced foods are designed to please the tongue and the brain instantly. This allows even a small quantity to trigger the old mechanisms of addiction that you will have broken on your Paleo journey up to that point. Therefore, it is crucial to understand that it will only take a few days of eating this junk to make you addicted all over again. With each new period of addiction comes another painful cycle of breaking it. So a failed day of

Paleo is fine. Three of four consecutive days over a long weekend could be a disaster for your progress in the long term.

Understand this and it will help you avoid the consequences and behaviors that began you on this journey to start with.

CHAPTER FOUR: TRACKING THE 30 DAY CHALLENGE

Why do a 30 day Paleo challenge? Why not just 'go Paleo'?

Some of the addiction to Western convenience foods revolves around habits. The habits that form a busy modern lifestyle. Although this is a health change, it is unlikely that the other areas of your life will be changed right now. Your job, your spouse, your kids - they will all continue to be a part of your life as they are. So the daily situations that constitute your existing mealtimes will need to be understood, changed and monitored.

30 days is a long enough period to break most bad habits. The daily repetition of an alternative, better choice will make temptation less and eating Paleo automatic.

In previous chapters, we've covered the reasons for going Paleo. Not only the health benefits, but also your own, personal motivations. We've also outlined the obstacles that will challenge and tempt you away from the change.

The final element to guarantee success is self-discipline.

Discipline is not as easy as most people think it is. Everyone believes themselves to be fairly disciplined, yet if you take the average of the people around you, then there is a good chance that their lives and bodies show no real evidence of the fact.

Most people don't understand the discipline required to complete the 30 day Paleo challenge. Again, it is not just about having a meal plan and a gym membership. It is about the daily monitoring that you put in place to understand, track and ultimately change the habits that keep you eating highly modified, sugary, salty – but tasty - food.

When do you eat the worst of the foods without it being a conscious decision? This is, after all, what a habit is. Donuts on Monday that the boss always brings to work? Take out on Friday when the week is done. Beer and a hot dog with the game? Chances are, you'll have done these things for so long you don't even think about them. Someone offers the box of donuts in your direction and you take one. Whether you actually want one or not. You might not even taste it as you return to your emails. The only reason you realize it has gone is because your hand is empty and you're licking your fingers.

Going Paleo will mean breaking these habits.

It is more than just saying no. A habit is another, older part of our Paleo brain. It means that we don't actually have to think about an action. This conserves energy and brainpower in case we need to look out for a wild animal stalking us. So you won't actively think about saying yes or no in these situations. It's simply: donut - hand - mouth - gone.

So the first step to a 30 day Paleo challenge is to plan and prepare for the habits of your day.

Habitual eating - meals and snacks

Take an honest look at your day and how you currently structure you food intake. It is best to do this for a full 7 day period, to cover weekends and recurring weekly social events. Don't just include the main meals you eat. Do you grab a latte on the way to the office? A soda with lunch? What snacks do you eat during the day to fend off the mid afternoon carb slump? The more you notice and accept about the realities of your current lifestyle, the less of a shock it will be when these things change.

Write these things down. You can use an app or a piece of paper. There are two factors that come into play when doing this. The first is that it makes you more honest and accountable to yourself. No one else needs to see this list, but you need to be honest. As you write it down, you will likely be surprised by how much there is that you need to change and how much you have been consuming in processed foods without realizing.

The second reason is that repeated research has shown that those who write down their habits are more likely to stick to them. The same works in reverse. By writing down the things you want to avoid from now on - the things you will *need* to avoid if you are to be successful for the next 30 days - you are dramatically increasing the chances of doing so. The more detail you write down, the better. Make sure you set aside the appropriate amount of time to do this if you are serious about completing a 30 day challenge.

Implement the challenge

The list you have created and defined above is now the main tool you will use to implement the 30 day challenge. This is the foundation for how you will integrate a Paleo diet into your life.

There are two routes to doing this. The first is that it will make you more conscious of the external forces that you have no control of. This, for example, is the boss that brings in donuts. Knowing they will appear means that you can be prepared to say no. You can take a walk away from your desk when the box appears. Or you can already be eating a healthy alternative, such as a piece of fruit, so the automatic response to put the donut in your mouth is inhibited.

For internal habits, such as the latte on the way to work, you can always ensure you have an alternative in advance. Prepare a healthy smoothie to take with you and when you pass your favorite coffee stand, you will already have a drink in your hand.

Switching to Paleo successfully doesn't mean that you simply eliminate certain foods from your life. For a sustainable lifestyle change, it is about finding the replacements and alternatives that suit you. This book contains a set of recipes you can implement to remove the need for on the spot decisions. That way you are never left with only poor choices or the alternative of being hungry and missing a meal.

Where possible, swap the bad habit for a better one. This may sound hard, but in reality, it is quite simple once you have been through the task of identifying your bad food habits. Do you take a break by heading down to the coffee shop? If so, then go for a longer walk instead, rather than waiting in line. Don't head in the direction of your usual route, but go the opposite way. That will break the habit. Setting yourself a target, for example, walking three blocks before turning back, will set a new routine that can replace the old habit and provide some additional healthy activity. It may not seem like much, but when implemented alongside the other, tiny changes, it all equates to massive positive action towards a stronger, healthier you.

Finally, track the 30 days and be amazed by the natural feelings of reward and achievement. Track it somewhere visible to you and make sure you clearly mark the success at the end of each day. There are countless habit tracking apps available for smart phones and a simple daily checkbox on paper gives an equal sense of accomplishment. The vital element is to have a visual representation of how many consecutive days you've completed of the 30 day challenge so far. It has been proven that after a certain number of unbroken days, sticking to the plan becomes a reward in itself. If you crave a burger and shake but know you'll break your 15 day streak by having them, you are less likely to do so as it means returning to day 1 on the chart.

If you feel that these methods aren't going to be enough to keep you on track, then join a support group. There are countless online groups that you can join by doing a simple internet search. Not only will these people cheer you on, especially if you are completely new to the world of Paleo, but they will also hold you accountable when the temptations present themselves. Like a sponsor with Alcoholics Anonymous, an online group can be global and therefore someone is around 24 hours a day to lend a helping hand along the way.

In these chapters we have covered the fundamentals for success that go beyond diet and exercise. So now you're set up to win, it's time to look at Paleo food, cooking and exercise.

CHAPTER FIVE: FOOD CHOICES AND CHANGES

The Paleo diet is easy to follow given that there are clear categories of allowed foods. If it is not on the allowed list, then you can't eat it and call it true Paleo.

Allowed foods:

- Vegetables

- Fruits

- Meats (lean, preferably organic/sustainable)

- Seafood

- Nuts and seeds

- Healthy fats

This leaves a list of banned foods that probably currently constitute a significant part of your diet. In a reversal of natural, healthy foods, they currently are the staples of the Western diet. Worst of all, they are generally consumed after being highly processed and modified, so are already removed from their original state.

Banned foods:

- Grains
- Dairy
- Legumes
- Starches
- Alcohol
- Any processed foods or sugars

Vegetables

It is only in the last fifty years that the Standard American Diet (or Western diet) has seen a shift away from fresh produce to packaged foods. In terms of human evolution, this is a shockingly small period of time and yet the change has been dramatic.

Vegetables provide countless macro- and micronutrients required for the human body to function at an optimal level. In addition, they have a high water, low calorie content, meaning you can eat them in abundance. Alongside meat, vegetables should make up a significant quantity of the food you consume when going Paleo.

There are only two caveats to take into consideration when you are choosing vegetables. Luckily, they are both easy to be aware of and recognize.

Firstly, it should go without saying now that the vegetables themselves should be fresh and in their original form. Do not buy vegetables that have been pickled, sugared, or in any other way preserved. These are the ones usually found in tins and jars. Pick your vegetables fresh from the produce aisles and you will easily avoid these items.

Secondly, although they are vegetables, items with a high starch content, such as white potatoes or yams, should not be included as a staple vegetable source. In terms of the nutritional value they provide, it is comparatively low when stacked against their natural sugar and carbohydrate levels. Eat them once or twice a week, but ensure they are not included with every meal as a replacement for pasta or bread.

Fruit

In addition to vegetables, all fruits are allowed on the Paleo diet. However, unlike vegetables, they should be consumed in moderation.

As discussed earlier in the dangers of pre-packaged

convenience foods, the fructose in fruit is metabolized differently from other simple carbohydrates. Given that our Paleo ancestors did not have access to fruit with every meal, then it shouldn't be treated as a freely available food source.

Everyone has a different goal for Paleo, but if it is your intention to lose weight, then fruit should be kept to a minimum. This is especially true of the highest sugar fruits such as bananas. If you are doing Paleo in conjunction with an intensive workout regimen, then greater quantities of fruit can be consumed as part of energy replacement and replenishment.

For the average person beginning Paleo, then two to three pieces of whole fruit per day is recommended as a maximum.

We would also recommend not eating fruit only in the form of juices and smoothies. Whilst delicious, the process of juicing introduces the natural sugars of the fruit into the body at a significantly faster speed than eating whole fruit. Depending on how it has been processed, it will also remove much of the fiber. The nutrient content may also be removed or destroyed. For this reason, if you do enjoy smoothies, try to ensure that a single piece of fruit is added for sweetness but stick to veggies to provide the bulk of the liquid.

Meat

Assuming you're not vegetarian, meat will be a staple food when going Paleo. As omnivores, humans have evolved over millennia to eat meat as their primary protein source. Sustainable, organic meat is the closest thing to Paleo meat, but it is not always possible to guarantee this. It can also be significantly more expensive, so may not be an option for everyone. However, if cost is a factor, then choosing real cuts of meat over a fast food burger is still the better option, even if it isn't organic.

Lean meats are the best, as they contain excellent quantities of protein but are lower in saturated fats. Although saturated fats are required and no longer as demonized as they were in the latter half of the twentieth century, they are not healthy in excessive quantities. Similarly, bacon, hotdogs, cured hams etc should not form the basis of Paleo meat choices as commercially prepared ones are filled with additives and preservatives rather than naturally smoked. If you're unsure, then check the packaging. If any sugar or other preservative is included in the list of ingredients, then it should be discarded.

If you're not sure, don't add it to the shopping cart.

As well as red meats, white meats such as chicken and turkey are allowed. These tend to be leaner than red meats, so give you a higher protein to weight ratio. Similarly, all kinds of fish and shellfish are allowed on the Paleo diet. This emphasis on protein allows the body to burn fat and build muscle effectively.

Eggs are a versatile addition to the diet. Not only are they delicious and healthy, they can be cooked in a wide variety of ways to liven up any meal.

Seeds and nuts

Obviously, if you have a nut allergy, then do not attempt to introduce nuts into your diet.

For everyone else, nuts are an excellent source of nutrition. They contain protein and healthy fats, making them a filling snack. They can also be added to many savory meals to add crunch and texture.

Nuts often act as an alternative to commercial, on the go snack foods. They are easily transportable and all taste different enough to provide a variety of flavor. If one of your pre-Paleo bad habits was frequent, between meals snacking, then keeping a selection of nuts available will help you resist temptation throughout the day.

Buy your nuts whole and unsalted and remember, the peanut is not a nut (more on that later).

The high fat levels do mean that nuts must be treated with caution if your primary motivation for Paleo is weight loss.

Seeds have their place too. As well as being another source of nutrients, many of them have a high fiber content. This helps to aid digestion and regulate blood sugar levels. Although no longer as common as they once were, seeds can be added to a wide variety of recipes to add texture and flavor. They also contain essential oils required for good bone and brain health.

Healthy Fats

For many people, actively consuming fat seems counter intuitive. For most adults, food industries and the media have pushed the low fat diet. This approach treated all fats as bad, whereas that is not the case.

Even saturated fats, once considered to be so bad that we needed to produce manmade alternatives, is required for the efficient running of the human body in small quantities. Avocados were once a serious no go for anyone attempting any kind of diet, but now they are so popular because of their healthy fats and other associated benefits that they are in constant demand.

Healthy fats are easy to find and are used as the primary energy source when available. This means that your body will utilize these fats efficiently and will only ever store them when there is a complete excess. Coconut oil is a fantastic alternative for cooking along with macadamia and olive oil. Nut butters can be used as alternatives to spreads.

For most people, the hardest part of consuming enough fat on the Paleo diet is purely psychological, especially if they have been attempting traditional approaches to weight loss for many years. But when combined with other allowed Paleo foods, it becomes easy to eat an appropriate amount to feel full, healthy and promote lean muscle mass and fat burning.

Seasonings

Seasonings form a controversial part of the Paleo diet, in particular salt. Salt is vital to the human body, but like many other things, consumption has dramatically increased with the adoption of the standard American diet. It is now widely agreed that the dangers of too much salt are high blood pressure, increased risk of heart attacks and strokes. However, a diet too low in sodium has also been proven to lead to health issues. So what is the right thing to do?

This depends on how serious you want to take your approach to Paleo. If you want to go true Paleo, then no added salt is a requirement. This applies to both table and rock salt. Even though rock salt has been less processed and therefore includes some trace minerals not found in table salt, the actual sodium content is roughly the same.

Even if you choose to go down this path, then the key is to ensure you are getting sufficient levels of salt from other sources. This means a high quantity of vegetables, especially leafy greens. You should be consuming this as part of your Paleo diet anyway, but with some people placing more emphasis on protein and fats than vegetables, it is a good reminder.

Another area that confuses people is whether vinegar is allowed as a seasoning, as this was introduced significantly after Paleolithic times and therefore wasn't part of the Paleo diet. However, vinegar is known to have health benefits and the finished product and its original form are the result of fermentation, a very traditional method of food production. Therefore, most people would allow vinegar as part of the Paleo diet, despite its relative newness.

All other seasonings are, of course, Paleo. Whether fresh or dried, they are simply plant product that adds a great amount of flavor without calories or carbs. As long as they are consumed in their natural state and not as part of a pre-prepared condiment, then they should be added as much as suits the individual taste preferences. So make your own spice blends and avoid ketchups and packets of seasoning which will usually have high quantities of added salt and sugar for flavor.

Additionally, it is worth remembering that many herbs and spices have been traditionally used because of the health benefits they provide. Science is now validating many of these ancient approaches and therefore you have nothing to lose by using them.

As you can see from the above, when switching to Paleo, there are plenty of food choices available. It is possible to take advantage of the allowed food groups to create a satisfying and varied diet. However, there are many items that are not allowed on Paleo. It is vital to be aware of these so they do not sneak into your meals and cause you to break with the Paleo lifestyle.

Banned foods

Grains

Possibly the biggest change you will experience in switching to the Paleo diet will be the absence of grains from your diet. This is a broad term for any flour, rice or corn based products. There are others, but these are the ones most often eaten on the typical Western diet. So no bread, pasta, tortillas, muffins, cakes, bagels etc. This can seem like a big change as they often form the basis of meals, especially breakfast. Grains produce an inflammatory response in humans, which can range from mild to chronic, depending on the person. It is one of the reasons why eating a carb heavy meal causes a bloating response. Many people find that in addition to common intestinal issues, skin conditions such as eczema and psoriasis are greatly improved when eliminating grains from their diet.

Dairy

Lactose intolerance is a term that people have become increasingly aware of. In reality, commercial milk is full of hormones and has been pasteurized to make it not laden with bacteria. In doing so, many of the nutrients are destroyed. The more intensive the farming process has become, the greater the amounts of estrogen in the milk we consume. This alone can lead to all kinds of reproductive and allergy issues, in both men and women. Many researchers have linked a high dairy diet with female cancers.

Although some versions of Paleo allow diary, for the 30 day challenge it should be eliminated entirely. If nothing else, this will allow your body to recover from a life of consuming products that were never designed to be consumed by humans.

Calcium is often cited as a reason for consuming vast quantities of dairy products. Good for teeth and bones, it is available in good quantities from milk and some other associated products. However, many vegetables such as kale or broccoli, or fish such as sardines contain good levels of calcium also. By ensuring you include them in your diet, you will still be able to maintain the recommended daily intake without resorting to dairy products.

Legumes and beans

Legumes and beans are excluded from the Paleo diet because, like grains, they contain gut irritants and inflammatory properties. They contain high levels of phytic acid. When consumed, this leaches away nutrients, meaning that even if you have a nutrient dense meal, if legumes or beans form the base, you will not get the benefits you believe you are.

Another gut irritant is the high level of galaco-ligosaccharides that are found in beans and legumes. These can be extremely irritant to people who suffer with IBS - the effects can be felt quite soon after eating. For everyone else, the irritation still occurs, but the effects can be milder. Like grains, they also contain lectin, which is known to produce an inflammatory response. Add all these elements together, and it is clear to see why the removal of these items from your diet will lead to a less sluggish, happier intestinal and immune system.

Artificial sweeteners

For many people, it is hard to justify avoiding artificial sweeteners. After so many years of consuming sugar and developing the taste for it, they seem like an ideal way to satisfy the sweet cravings and keep on track. When most people are still thinking in the traditional way of calories consumed, the fact artificial sweeteners are low or even zero calories seems like a no brainer when it comes to weight control.

However, artificial sweeteners need to be excluded because there is more to them than just their calorie content. They are chemical, man made products. The research into their long-term effectiveness and benefits to health has yet to produce any viable, unbiased studies. Without fully independent research, it is hard to know whether these chemicals could be doing the same damage, as we now know trans fats have been.

There does appear to be a correlation between excessive use of artificial sweeteners and damage to gut health. This damage then not only affects the amount of calories absorbed from food (making you intake and store more) but also weakens the immune system.

Some studies have even suggested that sweeteners can manipulate the insulin response and cause uncontrolled blood sugar variations, but at the time of writing, these appear inconclusive. Regardless, it should be clear by now that adding artificial chemicals into our systems are unnecessary and not worth the potential harm for the sake of a small amount of flavor.

If you have eliminated many other sugars from your diet and are only consuming low amounts of natural sugars from fruits or honey, then artificial sweeteners soon begin to leave an chemical aftertaste as your palette is restored to its natural settings. This makes them even easier to avoid in the long term.

If you do want to use a sweetener that is low calorie, low fructose, then opt for something like stevia. This is a natural byproduct and therefore doesn't break the Paleo rules. If a little hit of sweetness is going to keep you on track for the 30 day challenge, then this is the route to take.

So that is an overview of the food allowed on the Paleo diet, and the reasons why some foods that appear healthy are banned.

CHAPTER SIX: EXERCISE

Many people begin the Paleo diet as part of an all inclusive lifestyle change. This involves making the switch from not only a processed food lifestyle but also from a sedentary one.

The benefits of exercise have long been known. As well as muscle and joint health that you can see, it also promotes wellbeing that you can't. It is known to improve heart health and boost the immune system, both of which increase human longevity. The additional 'feel good' hormone hit can help with mental wellness and boost energy levels.

However, when combined with a Paleo diet, the effects on the body can become even more pronounced. More than just contributing to weight loss, the inclusion of exercise alongside a Paleo diet allows the body to become stronger and leaner.

It is important to note that Paleo exercise doesn't mean just getting a gym membership and learning to lift weights. It is about increasing the movement in your everyday life. The gym is a great place to get that extra motivation and access to equipment to make it easier, but it should never be the sole activity in a Paleo exercise routine.

Everyone about to embark on the Paleo 30 day challenge will begin with their own levels of fitness and these will vary widely. Therefore, this chapter does not contain a prescriptive workout regimen. It would be impossible to do so and an average approach would greatly under serve those who were true beginners and those who already have an exercise program they follow.

The key for anyone at any level is to remember the basic tenant of the Paleo approach: activate your body in the way that it was designed to live.

The Paleolithic body was nomadic, not desk bound. Movement was a constant and as a result, the human body is an efficient machine when exercised effectively. The downside of a gym membership is that it tends to promote intense periods of activity 2-3 times a week. This places an inconsistent pressure on the body, whether those periods are made up of strength training or prolonged cardio.

Many people believe that hardcore gym activity, five

or more days a week, can be as bad for you as no exercise at all. That is because no recovery time is built in, leaving the body exhausted. Cardio, especially, has been known to increase the body to a state of stress akin to the flight or fight response. When this becomes a part of daily life, rather than a genuine biochemical response, the stress on the body can actually increase the risk of heart disease, depression and a weakened immune system.

Instead, begin by assessing your own health and introducing some 'outside the gym' exercise to get a true picture of where your fitness levels currently are. If you believe yourself to be moderately fit, but struggle to climb five flights of stairs because you usually take the elevator, then you're probably not at the level you believe. Try to lift some heavy objects and see where your natural comfort levels lie.

Once you have an overall idea of your fitness levels, then begin to think of your body in terms of how it would move without the aid of gym equipment, vehicles or any other mechanical aids. This centers the thought process around natural body movement and away from bench press personal bests that isolate a small range of muscles.

Get into the habit of walking wherever possible. If you do have a gym routine, then don't see the recovery period as a time where you sit or lie down. Instead, continue with gentle walking or other activities that promote low-level activity. This will break the exercise/sedentary dichotomy.

Don't have a gym membership? That's fine. Your Paleo ancestors didn't do Cross Fit either. Walking and running can be done just about anywhere, for free. Pushups, squats, stair climbs, crunches are the same. It is about overall health, not creating a body builder physique. That may be a byproduct if you condition your body consistently, but it is not the start point or the end goal in itself.

As part of the 30 day challenge, if you are not currently part of an existing exercise program, introduce the following into your every day routine:

- Push ups
- Squats
- Crunches
- Jumping Jacks
- Plank (or modified plank for beginners)

Increase the number of reps and sets over the course

of the month, to make sure your muscles don't adapt to the exercise. Do them in the morning and evening, daily. This is a great level of exercise that will build muscle and condition your body, but without forcing it to the point where a long recovery period is required. Throughout the rest of your day, ensure you take regular breaks to walk and stretch, and avoid long periods of sitting. If possible, add a 15-30 minute jog or running session twice a week.

Sound too simple? Not enough to be real exercise? Try it. You will be surprised at how difficult it is to maintain this twice-daily activity for the full 30 days. Once you begin, however, you will feel the changes in your body by the second week. By the end of the 30 days, you will be ready to either increase the number of reps or be at a level where your goal is simply to maintain your newfound fitness.

CHAPTER SEVEN: EATING OUT AND SOCIAL EVENTS

It is unlikely that you will be able to spend the full 30 days of this challenge cooking for yourself. Doing your own grocery shopping and preparing your own meals is by far the easiest way to ensure you eat Paleo. It is also very difficult when spending time with friends and family.

The good news is, most restaurants will be happy to accommodate your dietary requirements, as long as you are clear about what you can and can't have. Obviously, a fast food restaurant is unlikely to be able to offer you any alternatives, so these should be avoided unless there really is no other choice. A handful of items may be Paleo, but the effort of making the decision probably isn't worth it. Other restaurants, where food is freshly prepared, should be able to vary the cooking process to make your food Paleo.

The key is knowing the correct questions to ask.

Asking them in a polite and friendly manner will go a long way towards getting the response you want too.

Most restaurants will not use a Paleo approved oil for cooking. Cheap, synthetic fats are most commonly used, or dairy based products such as butter. This means that anything fried or sautéed will automatically be off the list. Even a grilled steak will often be finished with a butter-based wash to give it that perfectly finished look.

This doesn't mean that you can't order them. Although most restaurants won't have coconut oil as a staple (although you can always ask and your might be pleasantly surprised), they are likely to have olive oil. Request that your food only be cooked using that and it will be as close to Paleo as you are likely to get outside your own kitchen.

Most restaurants are used to receiving requests for vegetables to be steamed, if they are provided in some other form. Many other diets, especially low fat or low calorie ones, advocate the steaming of vegetables to keep calories low and preserve nutrients, so this will not be a difficult request to accommodate. Side servings of vegetables are likely to be portioned in line with the standard western diet though, so it is worth noting that on a vegetable rich Paleo diet, two servings may need to be ordered.

Along with other common requests is for gluten free options. Many restaurants now have several gluten free options on the menu as awareness of conditions such as coeliac disease has grown. Although this doesn't guarantee the exclusion of grains and dairy by default, it may provide a firm base from which to modify a dish to meet your Paleo needs.

Salads seem like a natural and obvious choice for eating Paleo. Unfortunately, as many people discover, irrelevant of which particular diet they are on, the usual offering of salad is far from an untouched, clean plate of vegetables. Usually the dressing contains unhealthy oils, added sugars and an unnecessary amount of salt. Croutons and other toppings further deviate from making the vegetables the main ingredient of the dish. Shaved cheese is often added for flavor too. So if you order a salad, make sure it is a side salad, without dressings or toppings. It will be assumed by default that you'll want these, so it is important to be explicit with your server up front.

If you're going to a restaurant, look online for a menu. Most establishments have them. Check it out beforehand and find the closest to Paleo options. You'll be limited to very few choices but can eliminate plenty of options before hand. By making a decision in the comfort of your home, you'll be less likely to feel pressured to deviate when someone is standing waiting to take your order and your friends are ordering pasta.

If at the end of your meal everyone else orders dessert, then this can be the hardest time. Most desserts are heavily laden with either grains or dairy and are therefore off limits. A fresh fruit salad is the best option, but specify without cream or ice cream.

If you eat Paleo successfully at home, for the 30 day challenge and beyond, then the most important thing is to not undo that good work by feeling stressed and unhappy. Be as prepared as you can when eating outside the home and certainly don't be afraid to ask questions, but don't be upset and highly concerned if, despite your best intentions, things go a little off track. A restaurant may not fully understand the ingredients and will say something is Paleo when it is not. This isn't a malicious attempt to derail you. It is merely a sad symptom of how far from our food sources we have become and how little we understand nutrition these days. Very few restaurants fully cook meals from scratch; be as careful as you can, but understand that the commercial food industry remains beyond your control when eating out.

Of course, if you live in a city that caters for the Paleo diet, then the easiest thing is to convince your friends and family to join you there. That will save you from the hassle of questions and will also surprise them with how much tasty food they can eat. Many outside observers think that eating Paleo is the same as eating boring food, so it can be an excellent teaching experience if you're willing to share.

Fast food

Although being on a Paleo diet is diametrically opposed to the fast food culture, there are times when you will be faced with no other choice. The most carefully laid plans can be derailed by unforeseen circumstances.

With little option for variation and a high tendency to be pre-prepared, heavily processed food with the cheapest available ingredients, all fast food options carry a risk. However, if you find yourself with no other choice, then there are a few things you can do to get closer to Paleo.

Burger joints

Those who make their own burgers in house with freshly ground beef are ultimately more likely to be naturally tasty and of good quality. The better the quality of beef, the less need there is for added chemicals and seasonings to create a stronger and more pleasant flavor. The more commercial the establishment, the more processed the food is as a general rule of thumb.

With the growth in popularity of the low carb diet, burger restaurants are more accustomed now to requests for their menu items to be prepared without the bun. For anyone on Paleo, this is the first place to start. The bun is included because it creates bulk to a meal; without it, a single burger patty won't seem like much. So go for a double burger and request extra salad. Make sure to specify no ketchup, mustard or any other special sauce. Another tip is to up the available protein by adding bacon to the order. No fries if possible, but potatoes are allowed on Paleo as an occasional extra. They will be cooked in non-Paleo oil, but if you have no other choice, then this may be the sacrifice you make.

Fried chicken

As with all other fast food restaurants, the use of

soybean or canola oil is the real problem here. Otherwise, chicken is a great, healthy source of protein. The advantage of fried chicken over other, more processed alternatives such as nuggets, is that the chicken itself is clearly close to its original. Skin on, lightly seasoned is best. Over seasoned or breaded chicken is obviously not allowed, but the advantage of whole, jointed cooked chicken is that you can peel the skin off and with it remove the coating.

Although traces will always remain and therefore if you are intolerant to grains then there could still be a problem, but if you aren't, then this shouldn't derail your Paleo diet too much.

Unlike burger restaurants, fried chicken restaurants often have more to offer by way of sides than just fries. Opt for the salad and don't add any dressings or extras.

Mexican

Although it seems an unlikely option given its leanings towards tortillas and beans, it is possible to eat close to Paleo if you are willing to make some changes to the standard menu. There is likely to be some added salt and sugar to make up the seasonings and once again, the oil of choice is unlikely to be Paleo, but it is no worse than the other options above.

Guacamole will give you a good filling base. The less commercial the better, but the nutritional advantages of avocado are a great thing for the Paleo diet. Extra salad, meat and grilled vegetables make for a tasty and filling meal. Avoid any kinds of wraps, rice or bean bases.

Avoid:

- Sushi
- Thai
- Vietnamese
- Italian

These rely too heavily on non-Paleo ingredients to make up the main portion of the meal (grain and soy bases rather than meats and veggies) and removing them is either impossible or will leave you with nothing to really eat. It is not worth the hassle. Opt for another cuisine instead. Remember, this is only when you have no other choice and shouldn't be a conscious 'treat' decision on the Paleo diet.

CHAPTER EIGHT: HOW TO DOMINATE THE 30 DAY CHALLENGE

The next chapter of this book provides you with all the recipes that you will need to complete 30 days of living the Paleo lifestyle. Hopefully you have also been convinced that success over the next month relies on more than just knowing what foods are allowed or banned on the Paleo diet.

So what next? It's time to get fired up and ready to go. The next 30 days will be hard, but with the right mindset and planning, you can dominate rather than endure them.

Below you will find a simple step-by-step list of preparation techniques to implement, track and succeed where many others fail. If you struggle and find yourself giving in to your old diet at any point, simply return to the list and see where you went wrong. Then you can reassess and start again with a support structure in place.

1

Choose the day. This is the day you will fully commit not just to changing your diet, but completely embracing the Paleo lifestyle. Don't just pick tomorrow because it seems like a good idea. Check to make sure that you don't have existing commitments that will challenge your ability to stick to the diet in the first few days. If you are coming from the standard American diet then this will be a steep learning curve to begin. With time, it will become easier to juggle eating and exercising in a Paleo way with the pressures of modern living and social events, but the first few days will be tough enough on their own.

On the other hand, don't put it off until next month. Too far into the future and this will be another book that you read and didn't follow through on. Make sure it is soon. It doesn't have to be tomorrow, but make a commitment to start at some point over the next week.

2

Take the time to assess your current lifestyle. You may have done this at the end of chapter four. Understanding how far you are away from Paleo allows a gap analysis of the change you will implement over the next 30 days. The chances are that you will be further away than you would like. It will be easier to complete the next month if you are honest about them from the start. Don't just think about your meals, but also your exercise levels too. You will be trying to implement more movement into your day-to-day life. If you current week consists of TV dinners, then you will have many bad habits to break. More than eating different food, breaking bad habits will be the thing that determines your success or failure over the next 30 days.

Remember to consider the variations in your weekday and weekend routines. Be honest about any 'treat' or 'reward' behavior that you have that involves food.

Finally, take into consideration any mechanisms that already work for you when quitting something you've been addicted to in the past. I believe you should go into the 30 days with a focus on going 100% Paleo, but depending on your current dietary status, it is important to be honest and decide if you are going to start at 80% and work up to 100% by the end of the 30 day challenge.

3

Determine how you are going to keep track of your progress over the next 30 days. This is the positive reinforcement that you will need to stay on track.

It can be either digital or paper. The only requirements are that it allows you to check off the days when you eat Paleo and complete a level of exercise that meets the targets you have set for yourself. The more visual, the better. You want to do more than just tick a box and then have it disappear from view. You need to be able to see your progress and cheer yourself on when you stay on track.

If you can find someone else to keep you accountable, then do that as well. This is another way of tracking your progress, as well as providing some much-needed support. If you can't find anyone to partner up with in person, then visit online forums to find like-minded, driven individuals who want you to succeed.

4

Clear out the cupboards and buy the food you need to get started.

The recipes section of this book will give you a list of all the ingredients to turn your kitchen into a Paleo kitchen. But first, you need to throw away (or give away) anything that isn't part of the Paleo lifestyle.

That may seem dramatic, but many of the foods you have will contain addictive chemicals, designed to make you crave them. For years, you have been giving in to that craving. A combination of biology and habit will be stronger than your willpower to not have a small snack. Or one cheat meal. It will be easy to justify when the food is there in front of you. Quite simply, if it isn't there, then you can't eat it.

There is another, more subtle benefit. Most people will feel the financial pain of re-buying food when they threw or gave away the same thing just days before. When faced with it in the store, it somehow makes it more real that you are choosing to fail and that in turn stops you from making the purchase.

Even if you don't cook regularly, you are likely to have some dried pasta, noodles and snack foods in the cupboards. Breakfast cereals are in just about every household and must go. Any condiments other than seasoning should be thrown out.

With the store cupboard and refrigerator empty, it is easy to restock with healthy, wholesome Paleo ingredients. Then, when it's time to cook, you won't have to make any difficult decisions or rely on willpower to resist temptation.

5

This step has been proven in countless studies to help people stick to their diet. Not just Paleo, but any other diet that has been tested. Quite simply, plan your food for that first week. This not only gives you an indication of how much time you need to prepare, but also removes the decision-making on later days. After a few days, your body will begin to detox and with that comes the pain of withdrawal. When faced with making a decision at these times, your natural inclination will be towards the option that will give you an instant feel good hit. Instead, you will already know the next meal or snack, so won't be forced to make a painful choice.

When planning meals, make sure you include snacks too. The Paleo diet does not prescribe a set number of meals per day. Nor does it emphasis portion size and calories. But in the first week, you will find yourself automatically trying to eat to a routine and that will inevitably include snacks. So be prepared for them and decide what tasty, Paleo treat you will have each day in advance.

Alongside your meals, plan your exercise times and any days when you are going to do an extended workout session. This will help you stay on track and embrace both elements of the Paleo lifestyle.

Make sure this plan is visible at all times. You won't stick to it if you can't see it.

6

Paleo 30 day challenge: day one.

This is an important day, but it is far from the final day.

It is the day you have made the decision to change your life for the better. You are about to build a stronger, healthier you and be the best version of yourself. It's okay to feel good about that. In fact, it is vital that you treat the day with positivity because it is the start of something good. With all the external pressures that make living a healthy lifestyle difficult for the vast majority of the population, there will be many days ahead when sticking to the challenge will be tough.

At the end of day one, don't forget to mark off the success on your habit tracker. This is the first moment when living Paleo begins. You are now part of a club that has chosen to step away from the expected and instead focus on long-term health and wellbeing.

7

Your next milestone will be a full week of living Paleo. With seven consecutive days checked off on the calendar, this is the turning point for most people. If you get to the end of the first week, you are one of the few who are likely to manage long-term success.

You may have experienced some side effects as your body adjusted to a life free from harmful chemicals and added sugars. In fact, at this stage, you may still be experiencing some difficult changes, but know that the turning point comes very soon. Don't step on the scales, as tempting as it may be to do so, but notice that your clothes are already feeling looser. Depending on your physical start point and how motivated you've been, you may already see some changes in muscle definition. Don't get demoralized if you don't. There is still another 23 days ahead of you where the changes will become more and more visible.

Take time to reflect over the previous week. What went well and what was tough? From your meal plan, were there any foods that you enjoyed more than others? Perhaps there are new recipes you want to try?

Plan out the next 7 days, just as you did back in step 5. This will keep you on track, even though things will start to feel easier and more automatic to implement.

8

Days 8-30. This is where the real momentum begins. If you decided to ease yourself in to Paleo by starting at 80%, then this is the time you start to build towards 100%. By day 30, you should be living a Paleo life, both in terms of food and exercise.

Continue to plan your meals each week. Once you have completed 30 days, this becomes optional, but many Paleo advocates deem it crucial to long-term success in the face of never ending temptation.

You will continue to mark off your habits on the tracker during this time. The aim for a successful 30 day challenge is of course to make the 30 days consecutively. But if for some reason you have faltered, then do not give up entirely. Do not stop trying because of one small mistake. None of us is perfect and living Paleo is not to make you feel bad about yourself. It is exactly the opposite. So if you have a bad day, then begin again the next. Remember, better to make 25 days fully Paleo than to live all 30 filling your body with poisonous and addictive foods.

9

Day 30 - now what?

By day 30, you will be feeling the benefits of the Paleo lifestyle. For the vast majority of people, the worst of the withdrawal symptoms from excess salt and sugar will have disappeared. Many will already see significant changes in intestinal and skin health. You will have more energy and have discovered that the Paleo diet is easy to implement with a wide range of meals available.

With living Paleo becoming easier and more automatic, there is always a danger in becoming complacent. By now, the habit tracker will be part of your daily routine and there is no reason to stop this simply because you have completed the initial 30 day challenge you have set for yourself. It is completely normal to set yourself another 30 day challenge to stay on track. You are undoing the habits of an entire lifetime. 30 days will set you up for the best possible chances of success, but you will still need to make positive, conscious choices.

You may find that your support group, if you have one, is now more vital than ever for staying on track. In addition to keeping you Paleo, you will likely find that other people with the dedication and commitment to succeed will bring positive benefit to other areas of your life too.

Those are the steps to take in order to make the change from an unhealthy you to a positive Paleo lifestyle. These foundations will provide the basis for your success, so it is vital that you do not skip any of the steps. You may want to rush ahead and 'just get started', but this is not a fad diet that will last for the next month. It is a long-term strategy.

The second half of this book contains a tasty selection of meal choices to get you through the 30 day challenge.

It's time to begin!

PART TWO: RECIPES

In this section, you will find the recipes you need to successfully complete the 30 day challenge and go Paleo.

However, there are a few things you will notice that deviate from a traditional cookbook.

Firstly, there are no weights and measures unless they are absolutely vital to the success of the recipe. This is because being Paleo is not about portion control and calorie restriction. It is the exact opposite in fact. With your biochemistry and metabolic system returning to its natural state, you will learn to listen to your body in a new way. It will tell you - truthfully - when it is hungry and when it is full, based on your body time and activity level. You may find that because you are eating fresh vegetables and lean meats that you consume more than you ever have done before, whilst still losing weight and becoming leaner and stronger.

Secondly, because of this, there are no cooking times unless absolutely necessary. The time it takes to cook will vary greatly on the amount of food that heat needs to be distributed through, so depending on the meat to vegetable ratio that suits your personal taste, there is a risk that a prescribed time could leave meat undercooked. Therefore, always adhere to the standard food safety guidelines for meat consumption and ensure that vegetables are sufficiently cleaned before consuming.

Where recipes include some ingredients that are a gray area depending on how strict your implementation of Paleo is to be, this is denoted by a * after the recipe name. These ingredients have been included for added flavor, but can be removed as desired. It has been assumed a very small quantity of added sea salt is allowed, although hard-core advocates would disagree.

Temperatures, where given, are in farenheit.

BREAKFAST

Paleo Sliders

Ingredients
Portobello mushroom caps
Eggs
Bacon
Chilli flakes (optional)

Directions

1. Slowly cook the bacon in a large frying pan

2. Use the fat to cook the eggs in the same pan. Use egg rings or simply fry, depending on time and preference

3. In a separate pan, cook the mushroom caps until tender and heated through

4. Top the mushroom caps with the eggs and bacon, then add a few chilli flakes for heat (optional)

Recommendation: 2 mushroom caps and 2 eggs. Increase number of sliders as necessary for your body needs and exercise requirements

*Pumpkin Pancakes**

Approx 5 pancakes

Ingredients
1/4 cup almond flour
2 large eggs
1/4 cup pumpkin puree
1 tbsp coconut oil
1 tbsp coconut flour
1/2 tbsp arrowroot flour
1/4 tsp baking soda
1 tsp ground cinnamon
1 tsp ground mixed spice (ginger, nutmeg, cloves –
spices may vary by brand)
Pinch of sea salt
2 tbsp pure unsweetened apple cider
1/2 tsp pure vanilla extract
Any Paleo topping

Directions

1. In a large mixing bowl, whisk the almond flour,
    coconut flour, arrowroot flour, baking soda,
    ground cinnamon, mixed spice and sea salt until
    combined

2. In a separate bowl, combine the eggs, apple
    cider vinegar, vanilla extract, pumpkin puree
    and coconut oil

3. Mix the ingredients from the two bowls together to form a batter. Stand for five minutes to thicken

4. In a large skillet, melt some coconut oil over a medium heat.

5. Add the batter and cook until the edges begin to brown and the top becomes dry

6. Flip and cook the other side until brown

7. Garnish with a Paleo topping of your choice

Ham & Mushroom Omelette

Ingredients
Coconut oil
Eggs
Coconut milk
Chopped ham or bacon
Sliced Mushrooms
Sea Salt
Ground black pepper

Directions

1. Whisk the eggs, coconut milk and seasoning in a bowl and set aside

2. Melt a small amount of coconut oil in a non-stick pan over a medium heat.

3. Add the mushrooms and ham and stir fry until they begin to brown

4. Add the egg mixture and stir gently to combine the ingredients and allow the egg to begin to cook

5. Allow the egg mixture to set. Use a spatula to pull the edges of the cooked mixture away from the pan

6. When thoroughly cooked, slide from the pan and serve immediately.

Don't worry if you over-stir the mixture on the first few attempts. Ham and mushroom scrambled egg is equally as delicious! Recommendation is for 3 eggs per person, however this can be altered as necessary for your body needs and exercise requirements

Blueberry Muffins

Makes 6

Ingredients

1 1/2 cups almond flour
1/2 tbsp coconut flour
1 egg
2 tbsp coconut oil
2 tbsp coconut milk
1/4 tsp baking soda
1/2 tbsp pure vanilla extract
2 tbsp maple syrup
1/2 cup fresh blueberries
1 tbsp cinnamon
Pinch sea salt

Directions

1. Preheat oven to 350. Place 6 muffin cases in a muffin tray

2. In a large bowl combine almond flour, coconut flour, baking soda and salt

3. Slowly mix in the coconut oil, coconut milk, eggs, maple syrup, cinnamon and vanilla extract

4. Carefully stir in the blueberries until evenly distributed

5. Divide the mix between the 6 muffin cases

6. Bake for 22-25 minutes until brown and cracked on top. Insert a skewer to test – if it comes away dry then remove from oven

7. Cool on a rack before serving

Veggie and Bacon Scrambled Eggs

Ingredients

Eggs
Bacon (or ham)
Spinach (or kale)
Onion
Bell peppers
Mushroom
Sea salt
Ground black pepper

Directions

1. Chop the spinach, onions, bell pepper and mushrooms and mix together in a large bowl. Set aside.

2. Chop the bacon into strips

3. In a mixing bowl, whisk the eggs with a fork and season with salt and pepper

4. Using a medium heat, cook the bacon in a large skillet until it begins to release its fat

5. Add the chopped vegetables and stir through until they begin to brown

6. Add the whisked eggs to the skillet and stir until firm

Recommendation: Great as a breakfast on its own, or as a side to steak if going extra protein heavy

Big Sunday Steak Breakfast

Ingredients

Steak (organic, grassfed if possible, the cut of your choosing)
Coconut oil (or lard)
Sweet potato
Onion
Portobello mushroom
Tomatoes
Eggs
Bacon

Directions

1. Peel and dice the sweet potatoes into chunks. Parboil and set aside.

2. Chop the onion and add to a large skillet with the lard and cook until translucent

3. Add the sweet potatoes and sauté over a medium heat

4. Heat a griddle and begin to fry the steak, bacon, halved tomatoes and mushrooms, turning as required

5. Move the sautéed sweet potato and onion mix to one side of the pan and fry the eggs

6.   Serve and eat immediately

The timing of this will really vary depending on your individual steak and egg preferences. Don't be afraid to experiment a few times if it doesn't happen quite right the first time

LUNCH

Chilli Lemon Chicken Burgers

Ingredients
Ground Chicken
Egg white
Minced or finely diced onions
Minced Garlic
Finely sliced fresh red chilli
Lemon juice (to taste, approx half lemon)
Coconut oil (or lard)
Sea salt
Ground black pepper

Directions

1. Add all ingredients to a large mixing bowl and kneed together

2. Use a palm sized amount of mixture and roll into a ball. Flatten into a traditional burger shape. Do this until all the mixture has been used and you have your burgers

3. Melt the coconut oil into a large skillet over a medium heat and add the burgers

4. Cook evenly until golden brown on both sides.

5. Serve with a side of your choice

Caution: As with all chicken products, ensure the burgers are thoroughly cooked throughout. There should be no pink meat and the juices should run clear

Kale & Bell Pepper Frittata

Ingredients
Eggs
Chopped kale
Diced bell pepper
Diced onion
Chopped bacon or ham
Coconut milk
Coconut oil
Sea salt
Ground black pepper

Directions

1. Preheat oven to 350 degrees

2. In a mixing bowl, whisk the eggs, coconut milk, sea salt and black pepper until frothy

3. In a non-stick skillet, heat about a tablespoon of coconut oil over medium heat. Sauté the bacon, bell pepper and onion until almost cooked and the wilt in the kale

4. If ovenproof you can continue to use the skillet, otherwise, transfer the sautéed ingredients to a man and add in the egg mixture

5. Cook in the oven until the frittata is cooked all the way through

Recommendation: The frittata usually takes around 10 minutes to cook, but this time will vary depending on the quantity of food and the depth of the pan

Smoky Beef Avocado Burger with Paleo Ketchup

Ingredients

Lean ground beef (organic and grassfed if possible)
Coconut oil (or lard)
Egg white
Onion Powder (or diced fresh onion)
Smoked paprika
Whole avocado, sliced
Lettuce (whole leaves)
Canned tomatoes (drained)
Chopped cilantro
Lime juice
Sea salt
Ground black pepper

Directions

1. In a mixing bowl combine the beef, onion, egg white, salt and smoked paprika kneed together

2. Use a palm sized amount of mixture and roll into a ball. Flatten into a traditional burger shape. Do this until all the mixture has been used and you have your burgers

3. In a non-stick skillet, heat about a tablespoon of coconut oil over medium heat. Add the burgers. Grill until cooked evenly on both sides

4. Blend the canned tomatoes, cilantro, lime juice, salt and pepper to make the ketchup

5. Slice the avocado into strips

6. Top your burgers with avocado and ketchup. Wrap in the lettuce leaves

7. Serve and consume immediately

Spicy Garlic Shrimp 'Noodles'

Ingredients
Jumbo shrimps (tails removed)
Spiralized zucchinis (courgettes)
Diced bell peppers
Coconut oil (or lard)
Crushed fresh garlic
Freshly chopped chillis
Smoked paprika
Cayenne pepper
Finely diced onions
Sea salt
Ground black pepper

Directions

8. Spiralize the zucchini and set aside

9. In a mixing bowl combine the shrimp, paprika, chilli, cayenne, salt and pepper, ensuring the shrimp are coated thoroughly

10. In a non-stick skillet, heat about a tablespoon of coconut oil over medium heat and fry the minced garlic

11. Add the bell pepper and onion and sauté until the onions begin to turn translucent

12. Add the shrimp mixture to the pan and stir fry until the shrimp begin to change color

13. In a second non-stick skillet, heat about a tablespoon of coconut oil over medium. Add the spiralized zucchini and sauté until soft

14. Transfer the zucchini noodles to a bowl and top with the shrimp mixture

Recommendation: this works with any other shellfish if you prefer

Paleo Style Chicken Tacos

Ingredients

Sliced skinless chicken breast

Chopped chipotle in adobo sauce (buy or make your own)

Coconut oil or lard

Canned tomatoes

Fresh tomatoes

Sliced red onion

Scallions

Lettuce leaves (whole)

Fresh coriander leaves

Sliced pickled jalapeno chillies

Avocado (sliced)

Lime

Sea salt

Ground black pepper

Directions

1. In a non-stick skillet, heat about a tablespoon of coconut oil over medium heat. Fry the chicken slices until golden brown then set aside

2. Re-season the pan with coconut oil and sauté the onion until it begins to turn translucent

3. Add the canned tomatoes, chipotle mix and simmer until the sauce begins to thicken

4. In a separate bowl, mixed the avocado, onions, tomato, scallions and coriander to make a guacamole topping

5. Add the chicken to the sauce and cook until thoroughly heated

6. Add the spicy chicken into the lettuce leaves and top with the guacamole

7. Add salt, pepper and lime to taste

Chilli*

Ingredients

Lean ground beef (organic and grassfed if possible)
Canned tomatoes
Minced garlic
Lard
Extra-virgin olive oil
Finely diced onion
Chopped celery
Sliced mushrooms
Sliced carrots
Fresh, chopped parsley
Fresh thyme
Bay leaves (recommend 3)
Sea salt
Ground black pepper

Directions

1. In a non-stick skillet, heat about a tablespoon of lard over medium heat. Add the ground beef and fry until browned

2. In a saucepan, heat the olive oil over medium heat and sauté the garlic until it begins to release its aroma

3. Add the onion, celery, mushrooms and carrots to the saucepan. Cook until the vegetables turn soft, stirring frequently

4. Add in the cooked beef, canned tomatoes, fresh herbs, salt and pepper.

5. Slow cook on a low heat, testing for flavour regularly. Remove bay leaves or add more salt and pepper if required

Tuna, Avocado and Walnut Salad

Ingredients
Fresh or canned cooked tuna (depending on preference)
Avocado
Chopped walnuts
Salad leaves
Fresh sliced tomato
Sliced cucumber
Freshly squeezed lime juice
Sea salt
Ground black pepper

Directions

1. Add the avocado into a large mixing bowl with the tuna, lime juice, sea salt and black pepper

2. Mash into a rough mixture, adding more salt or pepper to taste

3. Top the salad leaves, tomato and cucumber slices with the mixture.

4. Sprinkle with chopped walnuts and serve

Broccoli & Cauliflower Fritters*

Ingredients
Coconut oil
Large eggs
Diced broccoli
Diced cauliflower
1 tbsp coconut flour
Grated mozzarella cheese
Chopped fresh coriander
Minced garlic
Fresh lime juice
Sea salt
Ground black pepper

Directions

1. In a large mixing bowl, combine all the ingredients and kneed until thoroughly mixed

2. Take a palm sized amount of mixture and roll into a ball. Flatten into a traditional fritter shape. Do this until all the mixture has been used and you have your fritters

3. In a non-stick skillet, heat about a tablespoon of coconut oil over medium heat

4. Add the fritters to the pan and cook until an even golden brown on both sides

Recommendation: If removing the mozzarella, then add more seasoning for flavour if required

Prosciutto Wrapped Asparagus

Ingredients
12 asparagus spears
Coconut oil (or lard)
6 prosciutto slices/strips

Directions

1. Cut the hard end off the asparagus stalk and wrap each spear in prosciutto.

2. In a non-stick skillet, heat about a tablespoon of coconut oil over medium heat

3. Add the spears and cook until the prosciutto crisps, turning occasionally

Sweet Potato, Chicken & Pine Nut Soup

Ingredients
Chicken breasts or thighs, diced
Diced sweet potato
Pine nuts
Chopped garlic
Extra virgin olive oil
Cumin
Turmeric
Paleo approved vegetable or chicken stock
Sea salt
Ground black pepper

Directions

1. In a non-stick saucepan, heat about a tablespoon of olive oil over medium heat. Gently sauté the garlic until it begins to release its aromas

2. Add the sweet potato, cumin seeds, turmeric, vegetable stock salt and pepper and bring to boil. Simmer on a low heat until the potato is soft

3. In a non-stick skillet, heat about a tablespoon of olive oil over medium heat. Add the chicken

and cook until it begins to cook. Add the pine nuts and continue to gently fry both until golden

4. Remove the soup mix and use a blender to puree until smooth

5. Add the chicken and pine nuts. Stir through the soup until evenly distributed

6. Add more salt and pepper to taste and serve

DINNER

*Hearty Sausage Casserole**

Ingredients
1 tbsp extra virgin olive oil
Sausage, sliced
Diced white onion
Cauliflower florets
Sliced carrot
Sliced celery
Diced potato
Canned tomatoes
Minced garlic
Fresh thyme
Fresh parsley
Bay leaves
Sea salt
Ground black pepper

Directions

1. Preheat the oven to 350 degrees

2. In a non-stick skillet, heat about a tablespoon of olive oil over medium heat. Fry the sliced sausage and onion until browned. Add to an ovenproof dish

3. Parboil the cauliflower florets and diced potatoes. Drain and add to the ovenproof dish with the sausage and onion mixture

4. Add the remaining ingredients to the ovenproof dish and stir until thoroughly mixed

5. Slow cook until the mixture thickens and the vegetables are soft

6. Taste test for flavor regularly. Remove bay leaves or add more salt and pepper if required

Pesto & Tomato Chicken

Ingredients
Sliced chicken breasts or thighs
Coconut oil
Chopped fresh tomatoes
Chopped sun-dried
Halved asparagus stems
Minced garlic
Fresh basil leaves
Extra virgin olive oil
Pine nuts
Sea salt
Ground black pepper

Directions

1. Create the fresh pesto by blending the garlic, basil, olive oil, pine nuts, salt and pepper

2. In a non-stick skillet, heat about a tablespoon of coconut oil over medium heat. Add the sliced chicken and fry until it begins to golden

3. Add the asparagus stems and cook for a minute before adding the fresh pesto mixture. Ensure asparagus and chicken is thoroughly coated

4. Add the fresh and sundried tomatoes and reduce to a low heat

5. Cook until the asparagus is soft and the chicken thoroughly cooked

6. Serve immediately

Spiced Salmon with Cauliflower Rice

Ingredients

Salmon filets (skin-on)
Cauliflower
Extra virgin olive oil
Smoked paprika
Cayenne pepper
Dried oregano
Chili powder
Garlic powder
Onion powder
Chili flakes
Sea salt
Ground black pepper

Directions

1. Create a spice mix by blending the Smoked paprika, cayenne pepper, oregano, chili powder, garlic powder, onion powder, chili flakes, sea salt and pepper

2. Coat the salmon in olive oil. Rub in the spice mix and leave to marinate for at least an hour. The longer the marinade period, the more intensely the flavor will permeate the fish

3. Blitz the cauliflower to a rice like consistency in a food processor. Add to boiling water for 1-2 minutes

4. In a non-stick skillet, heat about a tablespoon of olive oil over medium heat. Fry the fish on both sides until cooked throughout

5. Serve with the cauliflower rice

Seafood Alfredo with Zucchini Noodles

Ingredients

Scallops, uncooked

Shrimps (tails removed)

Calamari rings

Olive oil

Ghee

Coconut cream

Diced onion

Minced garlic

Chopped fresh parsley

Chopped fresh basil

Dried oregano

Spiralized zucchini (courgettes)

Sea salt

Ground black pepper

Directions

1. Spiralize the zucchini and set aside

2. In a non-stick skillet, heat about a tablespoon of olive oil over medium heat

3. Sauté the onions until translucent. Add the minced garlic and cook until it begins to release its aromas

4. Add the onions and sauté for 4-5 minutes. Add the garlic and cook for an additional minute.

5. Mix in the coconut cream, ghee and herbs. Simmer until the mixture thickens and reduces by almost half

6. Add in the seafood and simmer

7. In a second non-stick skillet, heat about a tablespoon of coconut oil over medium heat. Add the spiralized zucchini and sauté until soft

8. When the seafood is cooked, pour over the zucchini noodles

Paleo "Spaghetti Bolognese"

Ingredients

Lean ground beef (organic and grassfed if possible)
Spaghetti squash
Extra virgin olive
Coconut oil
Chopped onion
Minced garlic
Chopped tomato
Paleo approved passata
Italian seasoning
Dried oregano
Sea salt
Ground black pepper

Directions

1. Preheat oven to 400 degrees

2. Half and deseed the squash. Place on a baking sheet and rub with olive oil, oregano, salt and pepper

3. Place in the oven and roast until soft throughout (approximately 45 minutes)

4. Remove from the oven and put aside until cool

5. In a non-stick skillet, heat about a tablespoon of olive oil over medium heat. Add the onion and garlic until translucent.

6. Add the ground beef, salt and pepper and stir-fry until browned

7. Add the chopped tomato, passata, Italian seasoning and simmer stirring frequently

8. Remove the squash from the refrigerator and use a fork to create 'spaghetti' lengths of squash

9. Add the sauce to the spaghetti and serve immediately

Chicken and Pumpkin Coconut Curry*

Ingredients
Cubed chicken breasts
Pureed pumpkin
Coconut milk
Coconut oil
Diced onion
Diced bell pepper
Minced garlic
Chopped cilantro
Sliced red chili
Cashews
Sea salt
Thai red curry paste*

Directions

1. In a non-stick skillet, heat about a tablespoon of coconut oil over medium heat. Add the onion and sauté until soft. Add the curry paste, chicken, bell pepper, garlic, and salt. Stir to coat the ingredients in the curry paste

2. Add in the coconut milk and pumpkin puree. Reduce the heat and simmer until the chicken is cooked.

3. Serve and top with the chopped cilantro, chili and cashew nuts

Recommendation: If unable to find Paleo approved Thai curry paste, then swap for fragrant Asian herbs and spices

Slow Cook Turkey Casserole

Ingredients
Diced turkey breast
Coconut oil
Paleo approved vegetable or chicken stock
Ghee
Diced mushrooms
Broccoli florets
Cubed squash
Diced zucchini (courgette)
Minced garlic
Diced onion
Garlic powder
Onion powder
Sea salt
Ground black pepper

Directions

1. Preheat the oven to 350 degrees

2. In a non-stick skillet, heat about a tablespoon of coconut oil over medium heat. Stir fry the turkey with salt and pepper until browned

3. Transfer to an ovenproof dish

4. In the same skillet, melt the ghee and lightly fry the minced garlic and onion until translucent

5. Add to the ovenproof dish with the turkey and stir thoroughly

6. Add the remainder of the ingredients to the dish and stir until combined

7. Slow cook until the vegetables are tender and the meat is thoroughly cooked

Dry Lamb Curry＊

Ingredients
Diced lamb
Ghee
Diced celery
Diced onion
Diced carrots
Diced sweet potatoes
Red chilli
Minced garlic
Garam Masala
Turmeric
Fennel seeds
Coriander seeds
Coconut milk
Paleo approved tomato paste
Sea salt
Fresh cilantro (coriander)

Directions

1. In a large non-stick saucepan, heat about a tablespoon of ghee over medium heat. Add the lamb, onion, chilli, carrots and celery. Stir until the lamb begins to brown

2. Turn to a low heat and add the sweet potatoes, minced garlic, Garam Masala, turmeric, fennel

and coriander seeds. Stir thoroughly and cook for a few minutes until the spices begin to release their aromas

3. Add the remaining ingredient and bring to the boil. Simmer until the liquid reduces to a semi dry paste

4. Serve immediately and garnish with fresh cilantro if required

Recommendation: Serve with cauliflower rice or brown rice if on a cheat day

Fruity Pork Chops

Ingredients
Pork chops
Diced mango
Extra virgin olive oil
Chopped tomatoes
Chopped fresh cilantro
Apple cider vinegar
Ground nutmeg
Ground cloves

Directions

1. In a non-stick saucepan, heat the olive oil over low heat. Add the remaining ingredients and slowly cook until the mango and tomatoes break down, stirring frequently

2. Heat the grill to medium-high and cook the pork until browned both sides

3. Serve the pork chops and glaze with the sauce

DESSERTS & SNACKS

Chocolate Waffles⁎

Ingredients
Eggs
Coconut oil
Coconut milk
Coconut flour
Raw, unsweetened cocoa powder
Almond flour
Grated beetroot (cooked)
Baking soda
Honey

Directions

1. In a blender, puree the beetroot, eggs and coconut oil until smooth

2. Add the cocoa powder, coconut flour, almond flour and baking soda and blend thoroughly

3. Add the raw honey and coconut milk and pulse gently

4. Use in a waffle iron as you would with standard mixture

Banana Ice Cream

Ingredients
Sliced semi-ripe banana
Coconut oil
Almond milk
Almond butter
Honey
Chopped hazelnuts

Directions

1. Preheat the oven to 400 degrees

2. Bake the banana, coconut oil and honey until golden

3. Remove from oven and freeze for at least 8 hours

4. Add the banana slices, almond butter and a little almond milk into a blender. Pulse, adding the additional almond milk in stages until reaching the desired consistency

5. Serve immediately with chopped hazelnut topping, or freeze for later

*Pineapple Ice Cream**

Ingredients
Sliced pineapple
Coconut oil
Coconut milk
Almond butter
Maple syrup

Directions

1. Preheat the oven to 400 degrees

2. Bake the pineapple, coconut oil and maple syrup until golden

3. Remove from oven and freeze for at least 8 hours

4. Add the pineapple slices, almond butter and a little coconut milk into a blender. Pulse, adding the additional coconut milk in stages until reaching the desired consistency

5. Serve immediately or freeze for later

Hazelnut Ice Cream

Ingredients
Finely chopped hazelnuts
Coconut milk
Coconut cream
Hazelnut butter
Pure vanilla extract
Raw honey
Pinch sea salt
1/3 cup unsweetened hazelnut butter

Directions

1. Add the hazelnuts, coconut milk, coconut cream, vanilla, honey and salt to a blender. Pulse until smooth

2. Add the remainder of the ingredients and blend thoroughly

3. Add to the freezer and stir every thirty minutes until too thick to continue

4. Freeze overnight to fully set

*Carrot Cake Muffins**

Serves 6

Ingredients
1 mashed banana
1 cup grated carrots
2 large eggs
1/2 cup almond flour
1/4 cup coconut flour
1/2 tsp baking soda
1 tbsp coconut milk
1 tbsp coconut oil
1 tbsp honey
1/2 tsp vanilla
1/2 tsp cinnamon
1/1 tsp ground mixed spice (ginger, nutmeg, cloves –
spices may vary by brand)
Pinch sea salt

Directions

1. Preheat oven to 350. Place 6 muffin cases in a muffin tray

2. Grate the carrots and set aside

3. In a large bowl combine the almond and coconut flours, then add baking soda, salt, cinnamon and mixed spice

4. Using an electric mixer or food processor and the eggs and coconut milk to the dry ingredients until thoroughly blended. Add the remaining ingredients, including the shredded carrots from earlier and blitz until smooth. Add more coconut milk if the mixture is too dry

5. Divide the mixture between the 6 muffin cases

6. Bake for 25-30 minutes until brown and cracked on top. Insert a skewer to test – if it comes away dry then remove from oven

7. Cool on a rack before serving

Cinnamon Raisin Bread*

Ingredients
1 loaf Paleo Bread, cubed
Coconut oil
Eggs
Raisins
Coconut cream
Honey
Pure vanilla extract
Ground cinnamon
Ground nutmeg

Directions

1. Preheat the oven to 350 degrees

2. Lightly whisk the eggs, coconut cream honey, vanilla, cinnamon, and nutmeg

3. Melt the coconut oil into a baking dish to coat. Line the dish with bread and sprinkle over the raisins

4. Pour over the egg mixture

5. Bake until a skewer in the center of the pudding comes back clean

6. Rest for ten minutes before serving

Chocolate Brownies

Ingredients
1 egg
2 tbsp ghee
1 cup almond butter
1/3 cup maple syrup
1/3 cup pitted and diced medjool dates
1 tsp vanilla
1/2 tsp baking soda
1/3 cup unsweetened cocoa powder

Directions

1. Preheat the oven to 325 degrees

2. In a large mixing bowl, combine the egg, ghee, almond butter, maple syrup, dates, and vanilla until they form a smooth paste

3. Gently stir in the cocoa powder and baking soda

4. Pour the batter into a greased 9-inch baking pan. Bake for 20-25 minutes, until the surface cracks but a skewer comes back clean in the middle

Raisin Cookies⁎

Ingredients
1 cup almond flour
1/4 cup raisins
1/4 cup coconut oil
1 tbsp almond milk
1/4 tsp baking soda
1 tbsp raw honey
1 tsp pure vanilla extract
Pinch of sea salt

Directions

1. Preheat the oven to 350 degrees

2. In a mixing large bowl, combine the coconut oil, almond milk, honey and vanilla.

3. Stir in the remaining ingredients until fully blended

4. Line and grease a baking tray

5. Approximately 1 tablespoon of dough will make 1 cookie. When all the dough has been used, bake for 10-12 minutes until golden.

6. Transfer to a wire rack to cool before serving

Power Snack Mix

Ingredients
5 almonds
5 walnuts
5 cashews
5 hazelnut
Dried raisins
Dried sultanas
Dried apricots
Dates
Coconut flakes

Directions

1. Mixed the ingredients together and store in an air tight container

Recommendation: the above ratios contain enough for 3-4 average servings

Almond Cookie Bars❋

Ingredients
2 large eggs
1/4 cup coconut oil
1/3 cup maple syrup
1/2 chopped almonds
2 1/2 cups almond flour
1 tsp baking soda
2 tsp pure vanilla extract
1 tbsp almond milk
1/2 tsp sea salt

Directions

1. Preheat oven to 350 degrees

2. In a large mixing bowl, combine the flour, baking soda, salt and chopped almonds

3. In a separate mixing bowl, combine the eggs, almond milk, maple syrup, coconut oil and, vanilla extract

4. Combine the dry mixture into the wet mixture, folding until it forms a smooth paste

5. Pour the batter into a greased 9-inch baking pan. Bake for 20-25 minutes, until the surface

browns but a skewer comes back clean in the middle

Super Easy Nut Cookies

Ingredients
Walnuts
Almonds
Raw honey
Maple syrup
Unsweetened coconut flakes
Pure vanilla extract
Pinch sea salt

Directions

1. Using a food processor, finely grind the almonds and walnuts

2. Add in the remaining ingredients and gently blend until it reaches a dough-like consistency

3. With your hands, roll the mixture into balls of approximately one inch

4. On a lined baking tray, press the balls down until they take on a flat cookie shape

5. Turn out the dough onto a piece of parchment paper. Using your hands, roll pieces of the dough into small balls, about 1 inch around, and space out on parchment paper. After all of the

balls are formed, press down on each ball to form a flat cookie

6. Freeze for at least an hour before serving

Gingerbread Paleomen

Ingredients

2 eggs
2 tbsp coconut oil
1/2 cup coconut milk
1/2 cup unsweetened desiccated coconut
1 tbsp cinnamon
1 tsp ground mixed spice (ginger, nutmeg, cloves –
spices may vary by brand)
15 pitted and chopped medjool dates
1 cup almonds, soaked at least 8 hours

Directions

1. The night before, soak the almonds (or a minimum of 8 hours)

2. Preheat the oven to 300 degrees

3. Using a food processer, finely grind the almonds and desiccated coconut

4. Add the eggs, coconut milk, coconut oil, dates and spices until the mixture is smooth but sticky to the touch

5. Turn out the dough onto a piece of parchment paper. Use a cookie cutter to make the

gingerbread shapes. Dust with coconut flour if the mixture is too sticky to work with the cutter

6. Top with a little desiccated coconut

7. Bake for 12-15 minutes, or until the cookies are browned

USEFUL RESOURCES AND LINKS

Firstly, thank you for taking the time to read this book. I hope it has given you all the information you need to make the change to a Paleo way of living. If you have enjoyed this book, then please go to Amazon and leave an honest review. Doing so makes the book more visible to others and helps me spread the message of positive change.

If you would like a **free** downloadable workbook to help you through the step-by-step process outlined in this book, then go to the following link to subscribe. You'll also discover exactly which tools I use to monitor my progress and ensure success.

You can find more information on www.30daybeginners.com

If you would like to contact the author directly, you can do so at 30daybeginners@gmail.com

Made in the USA
Middletown, DE
12 October 2017